But You Don't Look Sick…
(and all the crap you wish people knew about your autoimmune/neurological condition)

Lisa Marie

Copyright © 2016 Lisa Marie

All rights reserved.

ISBN:1517720796
ISBN-13:9781517720797

DEDICATION

I would like to dedicate this book to my four amazing, beautiful, brilliant children, Liam, Grady, Emma, and Ashton. Thank you for always being a source of perpetual inspiration. I love you so much.

ACKNOWLEDGMENTS

I would like to gratefully acknowledge various people and groups who have journeyed with me in the years since being diagnosed with Transverse Myelitis. First, I owe an enormous debt of gratitude to my beautiful friend and writing mentor, Hilary Lauren. Secondly, I would like to thank Gina Hallam and Julie Parker for continually pushing me to be the very best version of myself, even when I've just wanted to throw the towel in (and also for bringing me copious amounts of Starbucks every time I get admitted to the hospital. You ladies are the best!). Thirdly, I would like to thank all of the incredible friends and supporters from The Transverse Myelitis Coalition and The "TM Folks" Facebook page. We have been on this bumpy road together. You all inspire me every day and your encouragement has gotten me through some of my darkest days.

Lastly, and most importantly, I would like to thank, from the depths of my heart, my beautiful family. Thank you for your unconditional love and support.

THERE ARE NO WORDS IN THE DICTIONARY TO DESCRIBE THE LEVEL OF FATIGUE I HAVE

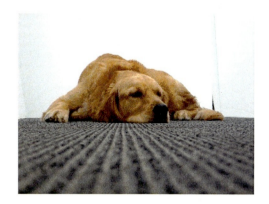

You've tried explaining it to your spouse, your friends, your co-workers, but there just aren't the right words to make people understand just how extremely tired you are. Like, "I've been up with the baby for 3 years straight, with no coffee, no sleep, and it's all I can do to stare at a wall right now" tired. So how can you really help people understand how exhausted it is just to be upright every day?!

Fatigue is one of the most debilitating conditions that people face with an autoimmune/neurological disease. It can significantly interfere with a person's ability to function at home and work, and is one of the primary causes of early departure from the workforce. Fatigue may be the most prominent symptom in a person who otherwise has minimal activity limitations. I mean think about it… your body is waging a war against itself daily! You should get a reward every day just for brushing your teeth!

So, here is what people need to know about your body and fatigue.

1. If I'm tired, I NEED a nap. I don't just want a nap and I'm darn sure not being lazy. Why don't we just let all of my white blood cells attack your body for a while like they do mine and see how you feel, hmm?

2. If I'm a little cranky, I NEED a nap.

3. If I ask you to repeat yourself 10 times or look at you like a deer in the headlights when we're talking, I probably cannot concentrate because I'm so drained… and I NEED a nap

4. If you love me, you'll buy me a travel pillow and blanket <3

I CAN TRIP ON AIR… SO WHAT'S YOUR SUPERPOWER?

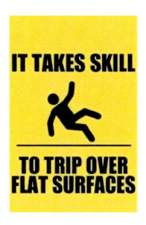

Getting harassed because your autoimmune/neurological condition has made you a little less than graceful? And where did that wall come from anyway? I get it! My husband tells me the song "Wobble Baby" surely must have been written for me. Am I insulted? No! I freaking wobble and you probably do too. I used to have such a sassy, cute gate… now my 9-year-old daughter refers to me as her cute, penguin Mom. That's always fabulous when you're in your 30s!

Here's what people need to know about your mad skills:

1. Uncharacteristic clumsiness is a "normal" part of many autoimmune/neurological conditions. Dropping things, being a bull in a China shop, and running into crap is just as obnoxious to us as it is to you.

2. If you notice my wobble getting worse, I'm probably being too prideful to let you know that I'm getting really fatigued and need to sit and rest. Be a dear, and make my butt sit down for a bit.

3. I know you like hiking, biking, and roller skating. I used to love those things too, but I'm not "that friend" anymore. I'm still a lot of fun! Like the super, funnest person to have a nice cup of coffee with ,or walk with… for like 2 minutes at a time.

THEY CALL ME DORY… HAVE WE MET?

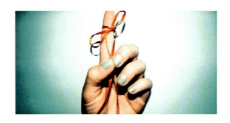

Where are my keys? Have we met before? Where is the peanut butter? What did I do with my favorite shirt? WHO PUT THE PEANUT BUTTER IN THE DRYER? Oh yeah… I may have done that. That explains why my favorite shirt is in the pantry.

Cognitive issues PLAGUE many people who have an autoimmune/neurological disorder.. Ya'll, this is just frustrating as crap! At times you may just feel like you're losing your mind; your friends and family may begin to wonder the same thing. Welcome to the new "norm". Just slap a dory t-shirt on and be on your merry way.

Here is what people need to know about why your toilet paper is in the fridge and you can't find the purse you just set down:

1. These diseases just really screw with your brain. It sucks. Don't yell at me or get frustrated that I lost my new sunglasses or that the milk went bad because I accidentally left it out all night. I was just as surprised as you were this morning when you found it!

2. If I ask you the same question five times, just answer it for crying out loud! I freaking forgot what you said! I love you and I promise I'm not just glazing over when you speak to me.

3. Don't get all high on your horse that you just beat me at Memory… my three-year-old did the same thing this morning.

4. Please just be patient with me. It's often embarrassing and extremely frustrating to feel like "50 first Dates" every morning when I wake up. I try to laugh off my forgetfulness, but a lot of times I'm left feeling confused and I just need some reassurance that it's ok.

"MAYBE IF YOU JUST LOST A LITTLE WEIGHT IT WOULD HELP…"

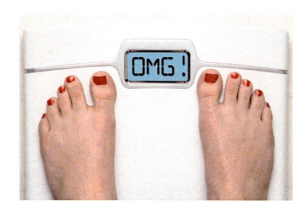

Are you kidding me right now? I live on steroids and rice cakes. Oh, and I can't exercise because my FREAKING body doesn't work! Ugh, I get it though. You get this disease you have and damned if you don't have to start shopping a few sizes bigger than you've ever been in your life. While eating a clean diet and staying well hydrated are VERY IMPORTANT steps in leading a healthy life, the simple fact of the matter is that weight gain is a common side effect of having many autoimmune and neurological diseases. Fatigue, steroid therapy, and depression can all lead to weight gain. Do not FREAK OUT that you are no longer a size 5! I haven't been a size 5 since the 4th grade… just for the record.

Here is what people need to know about the bigger, beautiful you:

1. DON'T freaking "let me in" on the fact that I'm gaining weight. I freaking know! And if you suggest one more time that I get a salad when we're out to dinner, I may throat punch you.

2. My EVERYTHING hurts, like 24/7. I'm not being lazy. I'm not trying to complain. I do as I can, which is much less than I'd be willing to do if I could

3. Don't think for a second that I'm just "comfortable in my skin" or "letting myself go." While I try to maintain a positive self-image, it's difficult to step on a scale or see myself in the mirror and wonder why I'm gaining so much weight.

4. Remind me that I'm beautiful. Not like, "Even though you're fat, I still love you." But more like, "You are really beautiful!"

DON'T MAKE ME LAUGH…I'LL PEE MYSELF

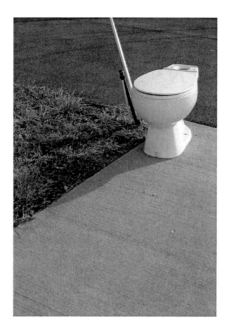

While many women that have had one or more children can relate to this as well, urinary and bladder control are common symptoms of many people who have autoimmune and neurological disorders. I have TOTALLY peed my pants on multiple occasions but am entirely too stubborn to start wearing "special undergarments." There's really nothing more mortifying than having a good laugh only to be left in a little puddle of fun when you're finished…

What people need to know about your bladder problems:

1. Nothing.. Some crap just needs to be private. If you're a pisser like me, suck it up and wear a pad the next time you go to the comedy club.

2. But if you're a really good friend… When I pee my pants, you just pee your pants too and we'll all have a good wet laugh about it. <3

DANG GIRL, YOU ARE SO HOT!!!....NO SERIOUSLY, WHY ARE YOU SWEATING? IT'S LIKE 60 DEGREES

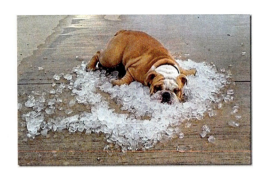

It's a beautiful 70 degree day. You used to live for beautiful 70 degree days. Now you fear any temp under 50 or over 70. Oh the joys of heat/cold intolerance. Nothing like getting all dressed up only to break out into a massive sweat as soon as you walk out the door or being bundled in wool socks at thermal underwear in the spring. Heat and cold intolerance are just another fun perk of having an autoimmune or neurological condition. When we get too hot or too cold, we experience a worsening of our symptoms, whether it be fatigue, joint pain, muscle weakness, or whatever.

Here is what people need to know about your broken temperature gauge:

1. My comfort trumps your comfort. If you having muscle weakness or can't walk well when you get hot, then we will re-evaluate. Until then, turn the AC on and all vents on me… I don't care if it's 50 degrees outside

2. My thermal underwear are sexy.. and so are my wool socks..and don't you let me forget it

3. If you see me sweating profusely, or shivering, please take notice and try to help me get comfortable, even if it makes you a little uncomfortable. I don't like to complain when everyone else seems comfortable with the temp., but it may really be hurting me.

"WHY ARE YOU SO MOODY?"...

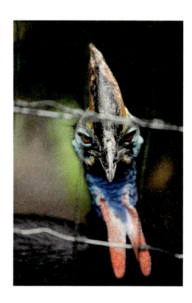

Moody?! What do you mean by "MOODY"? I am not moody! I'm just sort of sensitive… Dammit where are the Kleenexes!?

Unfortunately, mental changes such as moodiness and depression can ensue those affected with autoimmune and neurological conditions. Depression and mood swings can be the result of a difficult situation or stress. Being left with some crazy disease can be a very confusing and scary time. For those of us with demyelinating diseases, the disease can actually destroy the myelin that surrounds nerves that transmit signals affecting moods. Depression can also be a side effect of some of the medications we take.

Things people need to know about our Dr. Jekyll and Mr. Hyde moments

1. Don't tell me I'm being crazy….. unless you want to see me get really crazy. That doesn't help anything… and you make get a clock chucked at your head.

2. Sometimes I may lash out or get really down. This may be because I feel unwell, I feel discouraged, or this disease is taking a toll on my body. I need reassurance and maybe some space.

3. Watch my back for me, ok? If you think my depression or mood swings are getting out of control, it may be time for help.

WHAT'S UP WITH THE SPOONS?

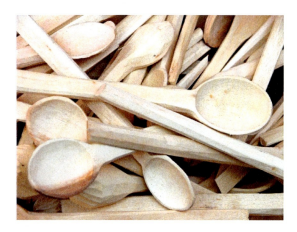

The Spoons are fundamental. If you do not know about the spoons, you need to know about the spoons. Everyone needs to know about the spoons. The Spoon Theory was birthed by Christine Miserandino while trying to explain to a friend what it's like to live with Lupus. She grabbed 12 spoons off of the surrounding tables of the restraunt she was at and gave them to her friend and said "Here, you have Lupus."

What your friends need to know about the 12 Spoons:

1. I have 12 spoons, no more. The spoons represent the amount of energy I have for the day. Everything I do costs me a spoon, sometimes more.

2. I do not have the luxury of endless possibilities. I have to consciously think about everything I do. If I need to go to the grocery store AND to the mall, I'll have to probably span that out over two days

3. Vacuuming costs me like 4 freaking spoons. I hate vacuuming for this purpose alone.

4. When my spoons run out, I can do no more. Even eating is too exhausting.

5. I will probably get a tattoo of a spoon

To read the entire story of the 12 spoons (and you must! She's amazing!), please visit http://www.butyoudontlooksick.com/articles/written-by-christine/the-spoon-theory/

YOU'VE BEEN EXHAUSTED ALL DAY! WHY AREN'T YOU SLEEPING AT NIGHT!?

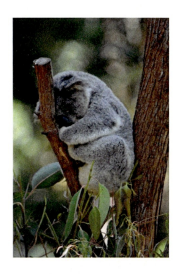

I've been EXHAUSTED all day and, lo and behold, the night comes and I'm the poster child for the Katy Perry song. You wonder how in the world I'm up when all I've done is complain all day about how I miss my pillow. Well, here's the deal, many people that suffer from this crap have go through the same thing. Sleep problems are common, and may be the result of a variety of symptoms such as spasms, urinary frequency, depression, or anxiety, as well as medications used to manage a variety of symptoms associated with the disease. (Oh the joys)

Here's what people need to know about your sleep issues:

1. Nobody wants to hit their pillow and sleep at night more than I do! I think I've broken a few world records in sheep counting.

2. Many people with my condition suffer from the exact same sleep problems. It's frustrating but it's common.

3. Sometimes I hate you because you can fall asleep before the lights are out. If I'm feeling particularly anxious, I may clear my throat really loudly in hopes that you'll put a reassuring arm around me.

4. If I'm single and sleeping by myself (or not sleeping) at night, be a good friend and get me a double dirty espresso if I'm looking a little rough in the morning.

DON'T ASK ME TO OPEN THE PICKLE JAR PLEASE!

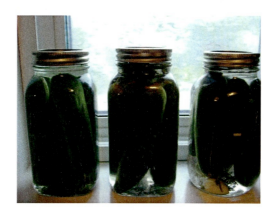

Oh how we used to be so strong and mighty!!! Pickle jar? I got your pickle jar! Oh but now…. we longingly look at the pickle jar, the jelly jar, the honey jar and wonder, "How will we ever eat?" Weakness can occur in those of us affected with neuro/autoimmune diseases which results from deconditioning of unused muscles or damage to nerves that stimulate muscles. So freaking frustrating!!!!!!

What people need to know about our pickle jar affliction:

1. I can't open the damned thing so can you please help?

2. My physical weakness is so frustrating to me. Please be patient if I spend 30 minutes determined to open the pickle jar only to start sobbing because I want so badly to feel strong again.

3. If you're a forward thinking, you can pre-open all jars when they come home… then when I go to open them, I will feel I will feel like Wonder Woman because I DID IT!!!!

FUNNY, THE WORLD WASN'T BLURRY YESTERDAY!

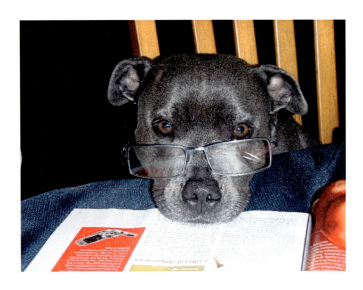

You've always been proud of your hawk-like vision but now you find yourself squinting to see the road and confused your Uncle Jim for your Aunt Jane. World getting a little blurry? Vision changes are relatively common in those affected with autoimmune/neurological diseases. Rarely do they result in total blindness but it's probably time to go see your eye doctor. A word to the wise, your sensitive eyes may not be thrilled about contacts so if you're considering contacts, get a trial pair first. And glasses make you look smart anyways!!!

What people need to know about your visual changes:

1. If I'm looking at the wall instead of your face when we are talking, I'm probably in denial about the fact that I need glasses. Go ahead and feel free to point out that I'm acting like Mr. Magoo

2. When I get my new glasses, tell me how super cool I look in them!

3. Visual changes can be scary, especially if I've developed something called Optic Neuritis (<—affects approximately 55% of people with MS) because that can cause double vision, blurry vision, and even temporary blindness.

DON'T TOUCH MY FEET!!!

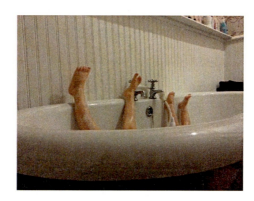

Remember those days when you loved foot massages and pedicures? Now the thought of someone touching your feet makes you cringe! The first time I went to get my toenails painted (not even a pedicure!) after being diagnosed with Transverse Myelitis, I kicked the poor lady painting my nails when she touched the bottom of my foot! I didn't mean to I promise! It was and involuntary reaction and I felt sooo bad. Many people with autoimmune/neuro disorders suffer from tingling/numbness of their feet. It makes it very uncomfortable when your feet get touched!!

What people need to know about your numb/tingling feet:

1. Don't get all bum-hurt that I don't want a foot massage. I appreciate the offer but it just feels weird to me now

2. If you touch my feet, I'll probably kick you… It may or may not be an involuntary reaction

3. Having sensitive/tingling/numb feet can be super frustrating. It makes it hard to feel what's under me and I can lose my balance. My feet get hot and then cold and then hot and then cold, making it virtually impossible to be comfortable so if I'm in wool socks one minute and flip flops the next, that is why.

Lisa Marie

OH MY ACHIN' BRAIN…

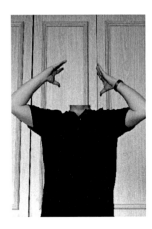

Like we don't have enough crap to deal with, our neuro/autoimmune disorder has graced us with frequent headaches. And by frequent headaches, I mean that some of us have them daily or some of us get them for a week straight with next to no relief from medications, oils, yoga, or whatever other "stuff" everyone advises us to do for them. Don't we sound like a bunch of whiners? Well, why don't we put your head in a vice grip for a week straight and see if you don't feel a little cranky about it, shall we?

What people need to know about your headaches:

1. I get them frequently. They can completely stop me in my tracks.. Yes, I've tried everything to make them go away. No, your voodoo concoction of oils and African wildflower is not going to help.

2. Because I get them so frequently I don't really complain about them, so if I do, it's a bad one. Try to be quiet and let me take a nap… or suffer the wrath of my crankiness

3. Headaches are a common symptom in people suffering with many neuro and autoimmune disorders. It clouds my thoughts and just adds to the daily pain I already deal with. They're not something I can easily work with.

I DIDN'T MEAN TO KICK YOU…I PROMISE

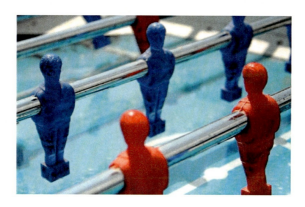

Oh that dreadful moment when your involuntary muscle spasms cause you to accidentally kick or slap someone… In my case the first instance was me kicking the nail lady painting my toes… and then I accidentally slapped my husband. (It was really and accident I swear!) He was a little more forgiving than she was. Involuntary muscle spasms are such a nuisance right? I mean, one minute you're sitting perfectly still, and then the next, your body is jerking in some weird motion and you've totally just freaked out whoever is sitting next to you…. Not to mention they can get really painful!!! These involuntary spasms, often referred to as "Spasticity" in the medical world, affect many people with neurological and autoimmune disorders.

What people need to know about our Spastic behavior:

1. I'm sorry I kicked you OK?! It's not like I can help it!!! Although I can't promise I won't use it as an excuse to kick some people… I kid! I kid!

2. When we go out shopping, let us avoid the China shop shall we? I would be what some may refer to as.. "The Bull

3. I understand if my involuntary muscle spasms kind of freak you out. They freak me out too. Please just know I don't have any control over it and they can be painful so just be aware of that.

Lisa Marie

THE ITCH YOU JUST CAN'T SCRATCH…

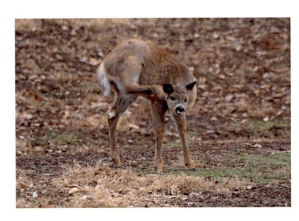

Ever have an itch you just can't scratch? How about having random itching all over your body that is never relieved by scratching which totally drives your freaking crazy every day of your life?!?!?! No? Well we have!!! Welcome to the FUNtastic world of Neuropathic Itching. (Can you sense the sarcasm there… if not, go back and read it with sarcasm) Mostly affecting those with neurological conditions, such as Multiple Sclerosis, this itching is caused when a transmission of nerve impulses cross sites where they do not normally occur and where there has been previous damage to nerves. That's fancy talk for "Our nerves are frayed and now we itch."

What people should know about your Neuropathic Itching:

1. I'm not carrying some weird, contagious skin disease. My itch actually has nothing to do with my skin!

2. If you see me hop up and start itching all over, I will throat punch you if your make "monkey" noises at me

3. As with many other symptoms I'm dealing with, neuropathic itching is annoying as hell, much more so for me than you so just shhhhhhh.

TODAY'S FORCAST...BRAIN FOG

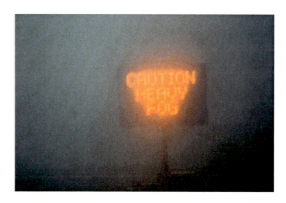

Out of it, Dream State, Spacing Out...... I've been accused of all of them! I can't tell you how many times I've been in the middle of a conversation and can't remember what I'm talking about.... or I set an alarm and can't remember what I set it for when it goes off. Sometimes I just feel like I just can't grab a thought in my cloudy brain!!! This condition is commonly referred to as "Brain Fog." Brain fog is a term neurologists use to describe a clouding of the consciousness, and is common in many people who have neurological, and some autoimmune disorders. This dulled state of awareness is often very frustrating and even embarrassing.

What People Should Know about Brain Fog:

1. If I appear to be spacing out, DO NOT snap your fingers at me! This is a sure-fire way to awaken the Brain Beast who resides in the Brain Fog and will give you a verbal face-slap for being rude.

2. It IS OK to gently remind me of what we were talking about if my train of thought seems to completely derail.

3. Brain fog is EXTREMELY frustrating!!! Like...sooooo frustrating... so please be super patient with me and love me even if I repeat myself 3 times... and love me even if I repeat myself 3 times.... and love me even if I repeat myself 3 times.

BACLOFEN FOR BREAKFAST…

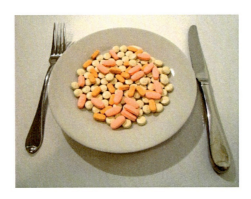

So my purse looks like a mini pharmacy… Let's not be so quick to judge ok? There was a time when I spoke the words "If I ever have to take more than three medications, just take me out back and shoot me." That was when I was "healthy" and now that's laughable. Nobody is more annoyed at the cocktail of medications I have to take every day just to keep me upright and moving forward than I am… let's just get that out there.

What people need to know about your bazillion medication bottles:

1. I'm not a "pill popper"… Well, I am a pill popper, but not the kind that you think I am! If you're wondering what I'm taking and why, just ask!!!!

2. Please do not throw your "If you just took cinnamon bark and root of witch hazel (or whatever)" in my face. If there was an "all natural way" to cure this crap I'd know about it and I'd be utilizing.

3. Although the medications are necessary, they're exhausting. I take so many pills in the morning, I don't even have room for breakfast! BUT… if I didn't have them I'd be in a lot worse shape than I am now sooo spare me your judgment because there's no harder pill to swallow than a friend or family member who refuses to try to be understanding.

SOMEBODY STOP THIS MERRY-GO-ROUND!!

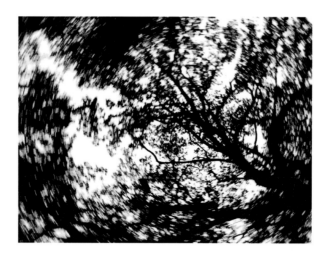

I'm just sitting here minding my own business in my world that is nice and still and BAM! Next thing I know my world is spinning and I didn't even get in line for the ride! Is there anything really that much worse than dizziness?! Just looking at a picture of dizziness makes me dizzy! Many of us dealing with autoimmune or neuro disorders get to battle it out with a little thing called Vertigo, or as I like to call it "Dizzy as Sh**".

What people should know about your Vertigo!

1. It can strike me out of nowhere so if we are out having fun and then I get super dizzy (and hopefully don't puke on you)…. do not make me feel bad for ruining a good time! Not my fault!

2. Dizziness makes it hard for me to keep my balance. If I'm clinging to a wall, please be a dear and help me get to where I'm trying to go.

3. It not a tumor.

BEING A DISABLED PARENT 101:

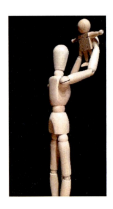

I'm pretty sure I could write a whole book JUST on being a mom with disabilities but I'll try to keep this short and sweet. Never in a million years did I think that smack dab in the middle of being a busy mom I'd get struck with some weird ass neurological/autoimmune disorder that would way slow me down. Like, my 5 year old doesn't even run away from me anymore… He knows I can't get around that fast so he actually just speed-walks away from me.. I still can't catch him. My 12-year-old knows that I have cognitive issues so he likes to ask me for something he's already been given because I can't remember that I already gave the kid $5 for whatever.. (In his defense, he always tells me he's just kidding and that I already gave it to him..I think…) SO, in the spirit of keeping my posts short and sweet:

Here's a few things to consider when dealing with Moms with disabilities:

1. If you come over to my house and it's a mess, and it will be, don't be all judgy! I managed to get my kids off to the bus with pants on and make breakfast that didn't consist of throwing pop-tarts at them as they bolted out the door to catch the bus.. the rest of my energy for the day will be spent on breathing.. and maybe thinking a little.

2. Being a parent is tough work even when you're healthy. Now throw in some debilitating condition and still try to feel like mom of the year. I don't volunteer for every field trip. I'm not on the PTO. I don't make every Birthday party. It's not because I don't care. I actually carry a lot of guilt over feeling inadequate because of my disability and whatever I have the physical capability of doing as a parent for my child, I'll be the first to do so!

GOOD DAYS AND BAD DAYS…DON'T JUDGE ME BY EITHER

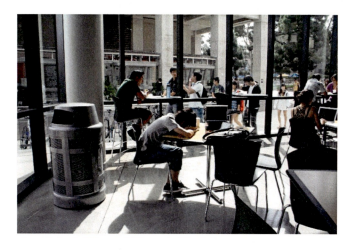

Some days you may see me happily buzzing around town with my kids or my friends and then some days you may see me pacing like a turtle in tar with my arm crutch, or even being pushed by my hubby in my wheelchair. Puzzled by the inconstancy of my disease?… well crap! So am I! All I know is that I have good days and bad days and I definitely don't get a choice over which days are which!

What people need to know about our good days and bad days:

1. It's next to impossible for me to make commitments to anything because I NEVER know how I'm going to feel.. So don't pass be off as being flaky or non-committal… I've just had to learn a lot about going with the flow… and there's no predictable flow

2. Don't assume because I'm up and about like a happy clam that I must be "faking" or "cured". I will 100% take advantage of wellness and am not "playing sick" when I feel well just so the world knows I have this condition!!

3. Don't assume because I'm in bed or having a hard time moving that I must be "hamming it up" either! When I'm down, I'm really down! I wouldn't be walking like Bambi on stilts for my own benefit! It sucks, ya'll. That's the truth!

I'M PRETTY MUCH A TOTAL BADASS…

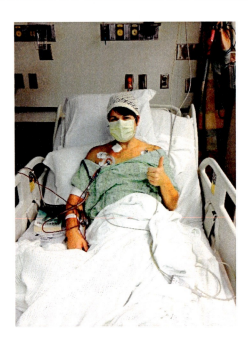

Commonly people with chronic illnesses can be looked at as "weak" or "fragile". You see this pic above you?! This is me with a giant tube in my jugular vein getting my blood sucked out of me, separated, and then put back in. Let me tell you, this is not for the faint of heart…or for the weak. Nope! Getting plagued with an autoimmune/neuro disease means getting to be a badass because ONLY a badass could go through all the crap we do and keep smiling and trucking along.

SO…here is what people need to know about just how badass we are:

1. Imagine getting poked and prodded, electrocuted, transfused, and rehabilitated from paralysis… Been there, done that… I'm a badass

2. At any given moment, I may not be able to walk… I may be plagued with severe fatigue…I may become very confused…. I do not live in fear because I'm a badass

3. I Refuse to give up… I will live life to the fullest no matter what my circumstances may be… I will be judged but I will have grace… and that makes me a total badass.

DAY 4…

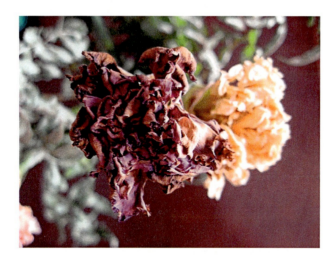

For many of us afflicted with an autoimmune/neurologic disease, that can mean long hospital stays. The first three days aren't too bad. You've got an influx of concerned family and friends, fresh flowers, and the hospital food is still appetizing. Besides, those first few days you're usually feeling too crappy to think about anything but just feeling better….. Then it hits you like a brick…Day 4. By now you've settled in, the first of your bouquets are starting to wilt and the flow of friend visits seems to slow down….leaving you feeling alone…and vulnerable. For me this means a good cry… I miss my kids, my soft pillow, my dogs, food that doesn't all look the same soaked in a brown gravy concoction..

So…Here's what people need to know about day 4

1. Day 4 may just be the beginning of my hospital stay. While you may think I'm "living the dream" in my hospital bed, I really just want to be back to reality

2. I'm emotional… Starbucks and chocolate are so appreciated… seriously…this poor excuse for a bad cup of Folgers they serve up in this place is enough to make anyone depressed

3. Come see me. If you can't come see me, try Skyping or Facetiming! I need to feel like I'm not alone in this and everyone's love and support is completely vital to my healing.

EVERYBODY POOPS…EXCEPT ME

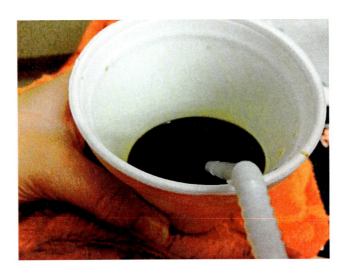

See that picture? Know what that is?! It's a piping hot cup of prune juice and Miralax. Mmmmm. Oh but we don't want to talk about pooping right?! Surely nobody can know how pooping, or the lack thereof, plays a big role in this disease process! That's too personal! WELL, I'm just throwing it out there… It's hard to poop… and at the age of 34, I never thought my bowels would be at the forefront of my everyday thoughts… but they are.

What people that can poop need to know about those of us that can't!!

1. Well, you really don't need to know about it… but we're talking about it anyways because we can't poop and it makes us grumpy

2. When I do poop, I get really excited! (My husband gets excited too) Like, it's a badge of honor in my house when Mom is pooping

3. Bowel dysfunction can cause a great deal of frustration and embarrassment for those of us with neurological/autoimmune diseases. It can also aggravate other symptoms. Just letting ya know! Raise the glass of prune juice with pride!!!

ANCHORED BY HOPE...

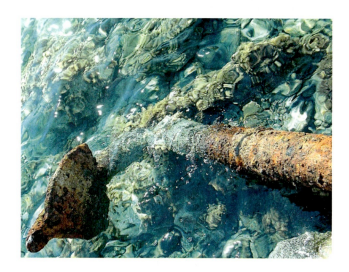

Ok, ya'll, we're gonna get real here for a minute OK? Yup, this one's for you! We've all felt hopeless, not that "I'm going to eat Ben N' Jerry's and cry for a little bit" kind of hopeless; but that "What good am I now that I have this (fill in the blank) disease? I'm just a burden to the world now" kind of hopelessness. I get it! I've been there... sometimes I still go there even though I try to anchor myself in hope.

So, where am I going with this? I was given a homework assignment by my beautiful friend, Julie Parker (who is a beacon of inspiration for me on both business and professional level) and now I'm passing this onto you!

What you need to do ASAP... NO procrastinating!

1. Download the app "iBethel"

2. Listen to Bill Johnson's Podcast titled "Hope in All Circumstances."

3. Comment below on your take-aways from what you heard!

I make no apologies for getting all mushy on you for a minute! It's good stuff. You can have hope! You are loved! You are a worthy person! OK.... back to the funnies

ALL I WANT FOR CHRISTMAS IS A ROOMBA

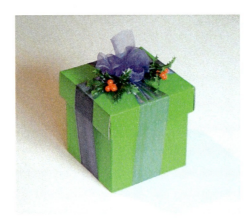

You know! A Roomba! That magic robot vacuum cleaner that cleans your whole house for you! Can I afford one? Absolutely not… Can I wish for one? Of course!!

Vacuuming is my least favorite chore of all. (and that's putting things nicely) With every swivel of the machine that would clean my carpets, it sucks my energy out of me like a ….. well….like a vacuum! A big horrible vacuum! When I look at my vacuum cleaner I become overwhelmed by the prospect of wasting all of my spoons on this ridiculous chore. It just sits there in all its dirt cleaning glory and smites me as I approach it, apprehensively, mocking me with its 12 AMPS of sand sucking power. Why oh why must we waste our precious SPPOOOONNNSSS?!

Ok, rant over… but seriously, here's what people need to know about us and vacuuming

1. I hate to vacuum

2. If I MUST vacuum (and I must…unless someone buys me a Roomba), I will probably need to nap for at least 3 hours and you can just forget about the rest of the house!

3. It's gosh darn frustrating to be faced with, what most would consider a daily task, with the daunting fear that I will be completely useless when I'm done. Please be super considerate of the fact that cleaning my house is a really HUGE challenge…

CANE SHAME…

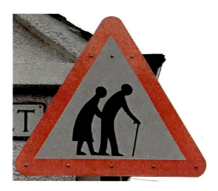

So there sits my walking crutch in the corner all alone. I know it's there to help me, and I shouldn't be so hard on it, but admittedly, I have cane shame. Cane shame comes when you go from being a yoga loving, jogging, paddle-boarding, sassy walkin' woman to a waddling mess, and need to use a cane to help you get around. Before my cane, I had swagger! I was a hip swinging, long legged, straight on the runway, sexy mamma! Now I'm a duck waddling, rubber band legged, stumblin' like I'm a drunk, swagger lackin' chick with a stick. It's a harsh reality for many of us. I'm supposed to use my crutch when I walk anywhere but I often just leave it sitting in the corner because I don't want to be seen with the stupid thing…… But I know that's unwise and prideful… Ugh… Those of us with cane shame must stand together (with our canes) and overcome! We must pimp out our canes and waddle with pride! We must not be ashamed of our canes but proud that we are still upright against all odds! Who's with me?! Anyone? Tap Tap Tap… Is this thing on?

I got fancy with the duct tape to decorate mine, but if you need a little help in the creativity zone, this is a great website with some sexy canes just for you! http://www.fashionablecanes.com/

What people need to know about your cane shame:

1. Hello, my name is Lisa…..and I have cane shame (everyone say, "Hello, Lisa.")

2. I know you think I should just be thankful I'm walking at all, and most of the time I am…but there are so very many days when I look at my cane with disgust. Why can't my legs just work? I don't want to look like a granny! I want my swagger back!!! It's just my reality!

3. I may look all sweet and harmless with my cane but go ahead and try making fun of me, it turns into a ninja stick pretty quick….so be kind…or hiiiiiiiyyyyyaaa!

YOU ARE ENOUGH.-THE MOVEMENT

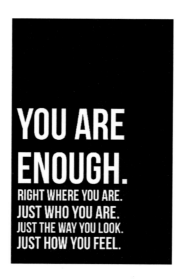

YOU ARE ENOUGH." is a concept that was birthed by one of my very best friends, Gina Hallam, and I. It's a statement that needs to resonate to all of us battling invisible illnesses. It's as simple as this. YOU ARE ENOUGH; right where you are, just who you are, just the way you look, just how you feel.

The term "Invisible Illness" encapsulates any and all medical conditions which cannot always be "seen" by others. Some examples of invisible illnesses include Multiple Sclerosis, Fibromyalgia, Transverse Myelitis, Depression, and a myriad of others. When we are struck with one of these conditions, it almost always encompasses to the feeling of not feeling like we're "enough" anymore. We feel that we'd be good enough if only we were still able to still do our favorite hobby, didn't have to take so much medication, didn't rely on loved ones to help care for us, could still work a regular job, (insert your "why" here).

This is a lie. We must stand together to believe in ourselves and to love ourselves wholeheartedly just where we are. YOU ARE ENOUGH. (emphasis on the PERIOD) Join us as we take a stand against the battle we face with our own hearts as those who are afflicted with invisible illnesses and know that WE ARE ENOUGH; right where we are, just who we are, just the way we look, just how we feel.

Peace and Blessings to you all, Lisa Helms and Gina Hallam

MY MEMORY IS GETTING SO......WAFFLES!

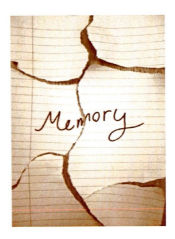

I know I've talked about it before but I'm talking about it again... I followed up with my Neuro a few days ago after taking a memory test because I'm fairly convinced my brain is turning into jello. My suspicions were confirmed by my Doctor, who just stared at me apologetically after I asked her for my results... That's never a good sign right?! And JUST for complete confirmation, as I was leaving the office she handed me a sheet of paper with the date of my next follow up appointment. As I was walking out the door, I turned and asked "Do I need to stop at the front desk to make an appointment?" Again... that apologetic look. Freaking waffle, sparkle, squirrel brain!!!

Here's what's up with our Dory brain ya'll:

1. I forgot

2. Just Kidding

3. Cognitive changes are a "normal" occurrence in people with many neurological conditions. It is a source of great frustration and often embarrassment. Yes, I will ask you for your name, even if I've known you for years... It is what it is. Please be so very patient with your friends with this issue! I may forget that we hung out last week, your birthday, or a favorite memory we had together. It's not because I don't care enough to remember.

WHEN YOUR WORLD FALLS APART…AGAIN

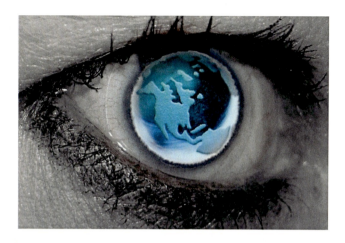

The first time your world falls apart is when you get diagnosed with whatever weird neurological/autoimmune disorder is; that you probably never even heard of before you got pegged with. You wonder how you will make it in this world. Why did this happen to you?

You begin making adjustments to your new life when BAM!!!!!… Your world falls apart again. It can come in many forms. Maybe you lose your job, your spouse leaves you, or your friends and family suddenly seem to disappear. You think to yourself, " WTF?! Like having this dumb disease wasn't bad enough, now I'm getting hit with this crap!"

Ugh, so annoying isn't it? The idea of trying to rebuild your life AGAIN seems like an impossibly daunting task…

Here's what you need to know when your world falls apart again:

1. When life throws you lemons, you pick those bad boys up and pelt them back at life with all of your might. You show life that you're not going to take its crap…or it's crappy lemons!!!!

2. Find support. If you feel like the entire world has dumped you, turn to a support group or FB page with other people who have your same medical condition. Rally up with those people and fight back!

3. YOU are a worthy person. You are worthy of stability, love, and relationship. As impossible as things seem right now, you've made it this far. That makes you a total badass and remember that. YOU WILL GET THROUGH THIS!!!! Piece by piece, and day by day, your world will start to take shape again. Hold tightly to hope.

SOMETIMES IT JUST HURTS TO BE ME…

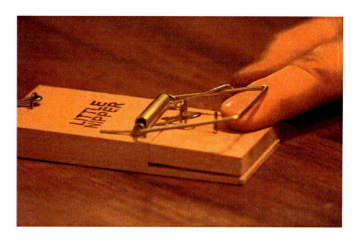

I'm sitting at dinner with a friend when all of the sudden I have a stabbing pain in my head. I'm talking on the phone with a client when it suddenly feels like I'm being electrocuted in my back, radiating down my spine and into my legs. This disease is so freaking rude! Many of us with neurological/autoimmune conditions suffer from intermittent or chronic pain. It's a giant pain in the ass… sometimes literally. Chronic pain can cause a huge disruption in our lives ranging from difficulty sleeping to severe depression.

Here's what people need to know about our pain:

1. So you want to know what it's like to be me? Stick your head in a vice grip for three days straight…. or stick your leg in a light socket…No? I wouldn't blame you. I don't want to feel this way either.

2. I try hard not to complain. I often smile through a migraine or attempt to do housework through debilitating back pain. When I do complain, it's because I hurt worse that my "usual" and a little compassion goes a long way.

3. Sometimes…well, often times, my pain requires that I back out on obligations or plans I've made. If I can't make it to dinner at the last minute, or have to cancel chaperoning that field trip, please understand that this pain is unpredictable and when it comes on, I can't help it.

WTF just happened?...

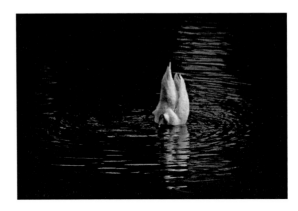

You're just making your way through this merry life when all of the sudden you are hit with some weird chronic illness that maybe you've never even heard of. In a matter of hours, days, and weeks your entire world is flipped upside down. You went from a daily regimen of a few multi-vitamins to having a pill box sorter for the variety of medications you take, half of which you cannot even pronounce. Your once completely active lifestyle has become sedentary as you learn to deal with new pain, fatigue, and feeling unwell. Chronic illness can take many forms. A few examples are Multiple Sclerosis, Transverse Myelitis, Lupus, Fibromyalgia, NMO, Rheumatoid Arthritis, and Diabetes. This just barely scratches the surface.

It hits you like a Mack truck, "WTF just happened?" "How am I supposed to live like this." "When is it going to get better?" These are all completely natural responses to the very confusing, and often times frightening reality of being pegged with a chronic illness, but perspective is very powerful. You can live with this stupid disease and still lead a fulfilling life. You can become a beacon of hope and inspiration to others. It's not an easy choice sometimes but it is a choice that only you can make. What will this "new you" look like? Will you be swallowed up with despair or will you rise up and show your chronic illness who's boss.

How do you go about this? Well, I'm no expert, but here are a few tips I've found to help me along the way...

1. Having a chronic illness is a bit like having a new baby without any of the joy that comes from a new baby. It may wake you up at night, prevents you from getting housework done, and exhausts you. Nap when you can. The dishes can wait. Re-prioritize. You have to put you first. Listen to your body and don't push yourself.

2. Do not feel guilt or shame for not living the life you used to. Maybe you went to CrossFit every day, prepared meals a week in advance, were in the PTA at your kids school. It's OK that you may not be up to or able to do those things. Learn to love new things. Maybe a yoga class might be easier than CrossFit. Cook but just one meal at a time and if you can't, keep take-out on speed dial. You can still be involved with your kids' school! Ask your kids' teacher if she has any work she can send home with your son or daughter for you to do, like cutting out pictures for an upcoming project, or sorting papers.

3. Don't keep your feelings tucked in. Talk about it, blog about it, journal about it…whatever!! Just find a way that you can safely vent, in whatever form you chose to do so

4. .It's OK to mourn the loss of the you before your diagnosis. There are times you will heavily grieve over the life you had and that's Ok. Just don't lose yourself in it. If you find yourself in mourning, set a time limit. "I will allow myself to grieve for 20 minutes and then it's time to stop." This allows you to acknowledge your feelings but not get lost in them. Go ahead and have a big, ugly cry about it! Then it's time to come back to reality and remember that you are still ALIVE!!!

5. YOU are a worthy person. You are worthy of stability, love, and relationship. As impossible as things seem right now, you've made it this far. That makes you a total badass and remember that. YOU WILL GET THROUGH THIS!!!! Piece by piece, and day by day, your world will start to take shape again. Hold tightly to hope.

Lisa Marie

ABOUT THE AUTHOR

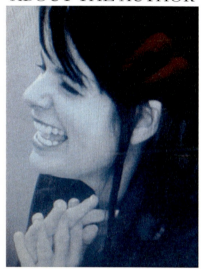

A nurse by trade, I found myself in the most ridiculous of circumstances when I got the sudden onset of a rare neurological disease called transverse myelitis in 2014. Forced to stop working (a "normal" job), I found myself frustrated because, quite frankly, I like to work. I started a blog called "But You Don't Look Sick (and all the crap people you wish people really knew about your auto-immune/neurological disease)" and found an outlet for my pent-up cynicism as well as a way to try to help bring some therapeutic laughter into the lives of others dealing with weird diseases that nobody understands.

Made in the USA
San Bernardino, CA
08 March 2017